DISCOVERING & TREATING THE FACET SYNDROME

Case Studies for 12 Medical Specialties

Discovering & Treating The Facet Syndrome

Case Studies for 12 Medical Specialties

2nd Edition

Nikolaos Giantsios

Orthopaedic Surgeon

First Edition: 2014

Second Edition: 2018

ISBN 978-0-9927821-3-9 (Kindle)

ISBN 978-0-9927821-4-6 (eBook)

ISBN 978-0-9927821-5-3 (Print)

Author: Nikolaos Giantsios

Editor & Publisher: Konstantinos Giantsios

Published by WTM News Limited

Office 4, 219 Kensington High Street,

Kensington, W8 6BD, United Kingdom

www.wtmnews.com

DEDICATION

The first edition of this book was dedicated to my family, my wife Olga and my children Fotini and Konstantinos for their ongoing support.

This second edition is dedicated to my son Konstantinos, for his perseverance and help to make it happen.

TABLE OF CONTENTS

DISCLAIMER

This book is designed to provide helpful information on the subjects discussed, encourage medical practitioners to consider additional potential causes of medical symptoms and to researchers a stimulus to dig deeper into the etiology of clinical entities which in this book are displayed as facet syndromes. The information provided here presents an analysis and interpretation of personal experiences and under no circumstances does it constitute the result of formal research or a guide of any kind.

This book is addressed strictly to qualified practitioners familiar with the spine approach. The information it provides is the outcome of application of the paravertebral injections for diagnosis and treatment. This diagnostic and treatment method can be tried only by doctors with surgical training who are familiar in handling emergencies and who are fully aware of the associated risks. The author warns practitioners and researchers that many of the ideas presented here require a high level of expertise and may hide significant risks. Medical practitioners are strongly advised to seek expert advice on any issues that exceed their education, training, experience and expertise. Spine surgeons could well be among those who would help them with the spine approach.

The publisher and author are not responsible for any health issues that may require medical supervision and are

PREFACE TO THE FIRST EDITION

When the mechanisms of automation in the human body get in trouble, the result is morbid manifestations to appear as clinical entities of obscure etiology. Their number is surprising large. Cases of this kind are enlisted in this book as facet syndromes since they were found to respond only when treated as such. A wide range of medical specialties are involved apart of orthopedics.

All facet syndromes are clinical entities well known to every doctor. What doctors cannot recognize yet on them, is their identity. This fact, combined with the lack of familiarity with facet treatment, is turning the whole situation to a major problem affecting a dozen of medical specialties.

The diagnosis of these syndromes is difficult, since they are displayed through channels of the autonomic nervous system. The latter, guarding its secrecy, provides limited only information to the examiner. This can hardly be considered as anything more than an invitation to solve a puzzle. Once the association between symptoms and facet joints is suspected, then the local paravertebral injections are those, which can verify them. The author hereby presents a plethora of such cases involving 12 medical specialties. They have all been treated successfully the same way, over a 45-year career.

Using the term facet syndromes, the author refers to a series of clinical entities, which are caused when fine nerve sensors, located in the articular capsules of the spinal facet joints, are in trouble. Similar sensors are also encountered in muscles, tendons and articular capsules of other joints. Certain of them provide information about posture and gravity, most important for the function of the kinetic and balance system. The irritation of these proprioceptors is the triggering mechanism for the appearance of the syndromes described in this book. The facet syndromes described up to now are related with the spinal pain. All of them are conditions triggered by the pain sensors of the same articulations.

Practitioners of various medical specialties come daily across these syndromes and are called to treat. The inability to diagnose them as cases, whose origin is the spinal column, is what makes their treatment difficult.

Cases of this kind concern dentists, stomatologists, ENT surgeons, ophthalmic surgeons, general surgeons, gastroenterologists, neurologists, neurosurgeons, urologists, gynecologists, rheumatologists, cardiologists and chest specialists. The orthopaedic surgeons are involved too, having the major share on them, although they do not suspect yet how far these syndromes are affecting them.

Their spinal origin was found first accidentally while treating patients with spinal pain, applying on them the paravertebral injections (PVI), a treatment technique widely applied in UK fifty years ago, with which the author is familiar. Patients treated this way, often reported back stating that other clinical conditions, from which they were also suffering and seemed to be irrelevant to their present problem, were also cured or showed significant improvement.

This unexpected outcome of treatment was in effect a trespassing of boundaries between medical specialties. Not surprising, patients belonging to these ill-defined areas are prone to meet difficulties when they have to decide who is the right specialist to treat them. A significant number of these cases are facet syndromes, which can be successfully treated if recognized as such. Their obscure etiology is what makes their treatment difficult. One can hardly detect any affinity with the spine. Most of them can present themselves at times with a different clinical picture that refers to a different medical specialty. As a result, wrong diagnosis and treatment is not uncommon with all the associated financial and social consequences to follow.

This book is addressed to medical practitioners of almost all medical specialties. The author is inviting his colleagues to rediscover with him this part of medicine believing that this new approach to certain medical conditions provides more effective alternatives to existing therapies. The thoughts and views presented here do not represent the results of a formal medical research process but a practitioner's personal experience as he systematically explored this domain over the past 45 years, trying to understand what facet syndromes really are.

The reader is encouraged to be inquisitive into the contents of this book and is reminded of the fact that quite frequently, what medical practitioners consider as experience and write it down, is nothing more than the repetition of wrong ideas adopted and practiced over time until effective alternatives are discovered.

The questions, which arise, further to what the author believes, should be discussed and answered by the medical specialties involved. The author, a trespasser in fields of foreign medical jurisdiction, is not authorized to do this. The reader is alerted that the treatment techniques discussed here hide significant dangers, which only highly trained and experienced professionals could be in the position to handle.

PREFACE TO THE SECOND EDITION

F our years after the first edition appeared, the author's impression is that it will take a lot of time till patients with facet syndromes will have the option of access to this kind of diagnosis and treatment.

The addition of syndromes not mentioned in the first edition and the further clarification of the expressed ideas is what this second one has tried to add and improve. What is particularly clarified, is that facet proprioceptors are accepted to be the sensors involved in the etiology of syndromes displayed in this book, distinguishing them from facet syndromes described up to now where pain sensors are the involved ones.

The upper fascia latae syndrome is entering this group as an independent entity or as a manifestation in sequence of the pes anserinus syndrome.

Pronounced forms of tennis elbow resisting to current treatments, were found to respond when facet treatment was added on top of the local one.

The Spastic Paraparesis case which is registered here as a lumbar facet syndrome, helped to recall similar cases from the past which in retrospect had to be accepted as facet syndromes too.

Although headaches are a frequent symptom triggered by proprioceptors, some headaches are differentiated here as a separate group since adhesions within these joints are considered to be the responsible ones.

Quite a number of well-known clinical entities are still waiting their verification as facet syndromes. Although some of them are insinuated, naming them was avoided. It is for the specialties involved to decide if they really are facet syndromes or not.

The feedback along the four years since the first edition appeared has revealed an existing hesitation towards injecting the spine. Quite probably, it has not been yet clarified enough that paravertebral injections (PVI) do not enter the spine canal, neither come across nerve roots. They are just aiming at the posterolateral aspect of the facet joints.

INTRODUCTION

The treatment of orthopaedic cases with medication delivered by the oral or intramuscular route proves quite often inadequate in bringing the desirable results. Only a small amount of the medicament is reaching the suffering site. Applying the local injecting technique, this treatment method proved much more effective for quite a number of clinical conditions. With this, sufficient locally acting medication is provided to the suffering area, protecting the rest of the body from undesirable side effects. The postgraduate training in UK at a time when the paravertebral injections were a widely applied treatment method, gave to author the opportunity to get familiar with it.

Upon returning to Greece, he started trying on the cervical spine what he had earlier learned to do on the lumbar one. He gradually realized that conditions, which doctors of other medical specialties were failing to treat, could be effectively dealt this way. The difficulties met by these colleagues, were due to the fact that the association of symptoms with spine was not known yet, and when one was suspecting such a relation he could not possibly know what exactly it was. With time and being continuously on the lookout for similar cases, he realized that this was a common problem for most medical specialties.

7

Many years later, when facet syndromes started being discussed, the author came to realize that what he was treating all these years were facet syndromes too, due to a different kind of sensors. With this term one is referred to various clinical conditions, which are the result of irritation of nerve sensors encountered in the capsules of the spinal facet joints. It was much later when it was realized that orthopaedic surgeons had the same difficulties too and that many of their obscure diagnostic problems are facet syndromes. Being preoccupied with current beliefs was certainly one of the reasons. The fact that bone vascular changes were not early detectable on the ordinary X-R films was another one.

Today, MRI reports detect from the start blood supply interference and impending or established bone necrosis. They still cannot verify if an intraosseous vascular change is reversible or not, neither confirm if there are bone cells still alive. Furthermore, they cannot point out any connection with the facets. The diagnosis of a facet syndrome in the author's days was purely clinical. Quite probably, it still is.

All cases reported here belong to the above-mentioned specialties. The decision to classify them as facet syndromes was based on the fact that they could be cured only when the involved facets joints were treated first. For organization purposes, an informal classification has been applied according to the location of the related facets on the spine. The gross interpretations given while discussing each case were inevitable. They reveal the way the author was trying to understand them.

This book is not the result of a formal medical research process even though a systematic pursuit was followed but merely a presentation of personal experiences as they all matured in mind over a 45-year career. Using representative cases was a convenient way for the author to display his beliefs.

Background Knowledge

"Facet Syndromes" is a specific term for clinical entities, which have as origin the posterior intervertebral articulations. The term "Cervical Syndromes" was a common term for most of them. Apart of them, thirty or more well known clinical entities, covering a dozen of medical specialties are now added to this group believed to be facet syndromes too. They were verified as such while treating the spinal pain with the local injecting technique.

Suffering posterior intervertebral articulations, known as facet joints, are focused to be the site where these syndromes start. The articular capsules of these joints host a rich network of fine nerve fibers, each one serving a certain function. The *pain sensors* are those, which inform the cortex for any facet problem, which follows trauma or mechanical strain. They are similar to the pain sensors encountered in any peripheral joint and their role is to display the spine problem as a local or radiating pain. They are responsible for the early phase of a facet syndrome, which is a reversible one.

Some other sensors of the same facet joints are suffering too. These are the *proprioceptors,* which provide information to the balance center, about posture and gravity. Similar sensors are also encountered in tendons, muscles, ligaments and capsules of other peripheral joints serving the same purpose. All of them are serving the autonomic nervous system (ANS). Inwards information arrives to the balance center from other sensory systems too, like vision and hearing, which are also on line

9

connected with the balance system. It appears that the information the proprioceptors send, is shared by all these collaborating systems, otherwise the balance system could not work.

In an instant danger for example, both hearing and vision are participating. The stereoscopic hearing is the one, which recognizes the direction of the oncoming threat and vision the one who checks the landing site if a jump away is decided. This has to be compatible with gravity. These two systems could not possibly cooperate with the kinetic and balance system, if they had not received from proprioceptors the same information about posture and gravity, which the rest of the participants had. This implies, that at any given moment, online communication is available to these sensors to send when in trouble their distress signals to all of them. It is the vasomotor center of any one of these systems the one which will finally be triggered to respond affecting organs of the system it serves. The result will be the appearance of the late phase of a facet syndrome added to the early one when vessels nerves and organs start being affected. This can be reversed at its early stage only before any irreversible lesions have been established.

In other words the problem of the suffering intervertebral articulations is projected as a problem of an otherwise healthy till that moment system, whose vasomotor center was triggered to respond to a petition for help.

> *"The triangle of interactions which lead to a facet syndrome of this group is drawn between a **suffering facet joint** where the stimulus is born, a **vasomotor center** which is triggered to respond and a **target organ** which is finally affected."*

Looking at facet syndromes this way, one can understand them as the substitute of a missing communication language between the two nervous systems. They are in effect some kind of a primitive language, which the body's administration, the ANS, has decided to adopt in order to remind the cortex for problems of his responsibility.

This language is displayed at the start with smoke signals, which are a local or referred pain addressed to the cortex. It is the pain sensors those who are doing this. When the cortex has repeatedly ignored these signals which are informing him that spine is suffering, then comes the turn of vasomotor centers, which responding to the distress signals which the proprioceptors keep sending to them, proceed to peripheral vasomotor reactions.

This is the time when sacrifices start. Diagnosing the facet syndromes is a decoding process on this primitive language, which has remained the same all along the evolution time for the sake of our survival. Quite probably, the ANS (administration) has decided that it is much safer if the cortex is kept out when quick decisions concerning survival have to be taken.

Since vision and hearing are close partners of the kinetic and balance system, they cannot possibly be immune of facet's interference. Distress signals from facet proprioceptors are reaching them too. Their vasomotor centers might be triggered to respond.

The author's belief is that a lot of the problems the Ophthalmologists and ENT surgeons come across are facet syndromes. These are entities whose obscure etiology is still considered to be an unidentified central one. The involved specialists are dealing with the peripheral problem not suspecting that facet joints are those who stand behind the central one. He had to adopt this concept trying to explain conditions, which he, by coincidence had come across and helped, although this was not his original intention.

Deep fascia structures are target organs, which concern the orthopaedic surgeons. Tendons and thickened straps of deep fascia are parts of it. The muscles themselves are indirectly affected through these structures. The overlying superficial fascia can be affected too. Soft tissue therapists who deal with them could offer much more to their clients if doctors had treated facet joints and local inflammation first before referring these patients to them.

More than one of medical specialties can be involved in the same clinical picture. This happens when vasomotor centers of more than one system will be triggered to respond the same time or in sequence.

> *"This way, the same facets can each time project their problem under a different clinical picture, and the same clinical picture can each time be triggered by different facets."*

This happens because proprioceptors of all facet joints, no matter how remote they are, have theoretically equal rights of access to vasomotor centers of any system affiliated to the balance center. The information they provide is equally important to all of them.

Tracing and treating the involved facets are abilities, which the practitioner has to develop in order to verify and then treat a facet syndrome. This is achieved gradually. His adequacy will never stop being tested.

This whole concept is an empirical one and derives from the fact that things return to normal only when the responsible facet joints have received the treatment they need. It is the result of treatment, what verifies a facet syndrome. This fact is reversing the usual sequence in medical practice, where doctors are diagnosing first and then proceed with treatment. This is a luxury, which the one who treats these syndromes, will never have. He is allowed only to suspect them first, having to rely upon his clinical estimation and then to proceed with treatment. The diagnosis is verified last, by the result of treatment. The saying "you can't argue with success" finds its application here.

What is comforting is that the triggering mechanism, which starts and maintains these syndromes, stops immediately after the right facets have been treated. This leaves no room for doubts about what one is treating, neither time enough for obsessions to be built since the answer, when positive, is either immediate or can take a couple of days. Restoration to normal is achieved when this treatment is provided timely, before any irreversible vascular changes have destroyed nerves and organs.

THE START OF A JOURNEY

I t was in February 1962 when the author started a three months training course as an overseas postgraduate student at the Royal National Orthopaedic Hospital in London. This was his introductory course on British Orthopaedics before starting applying for jobs, which would provide to him the training he was aiming to. His only previous experience was the 18-month training he had as an SHO at the Children's Orthopaedic Hospital in Penteli near Athens, which had provided to him a lot of surgical experience on children's orthopaedics.

This was the start of an Odyssey through totally six hospitals in UK. The British postgraduate training system demanded from specializing doctors to move from hospital to hospital up to the end of their training. The appointments of an SHO lasted one year, while those of Registrars a maximum of two. In other words, the British applied in training what Homer believed 3.000 years ago to have added on Ulysses' wisdom as *"he had visited the cities of many people and understood their way of thinking"*.

The training consisted of attending lectures, ward rounds, theater operations and outpatient clinics. The admitted, by the various consultants patients, were attended by the same nursing and medical staff. The doctors under training were attending patients of more than one consultant whose approach to medical problems might differ.

The consultants, representing the British Orthopaedic Institute, were among the eminent. They were the kind of pioneers who were striving for something new. The final message was that medicine is continuously evolving and everybody should understand that he is involved in this process. This was actually the start of the most interesting period of his career realizing that absolute knowledge does not exist. No one could hand down omniscient experience; instead he had to build up his own beliefs without the luxury of adopting ideas and practices unchallenged.

This actually started in May 1962 with his first appointment as an SHO at the Royal Hospital in Chesterfield, a small town of Derbyshire in Midlands. The orthopedic department was a relatively small one of 45 beds, with two consultants, one registrar and one SHO.

It is evident that in a reversed pyramid system like this, all the supporting work was shared between Registrar and SHO in a way that a heavy week of 127 hours was followed by a lighter one of 96. Their abilities were rewarded, by being entrusted with more responsible work. This heavy schedule was accepted as a fast track training course. This rhythm continued more or less the same with the appointments, which followed. Strange enough this tough five years period is recalled among the best. This was a period he had really enjoyed adding knowledge.

On the fifth month of this appointment, he was the one left to get in charge of the Injection Clinic, since the pressing waiting list moved the registrar in charge to theater work. Every Wednesday, between 2pm and 5pm, a number of 15 to 25 outpatients with joint and spinal problems referred by consultants should be looked after. The paravertebral injections (P.V.I.) to the lower spine were common practice. He was given the proper instructions and was left alone to his own devices. This continued for the next seven months until the end of his appointment.

As an experience, it was terrific. It was quite a challenge to get familiar in approaching almost any part of the skeleton with a needle, blindly, without any technical localizing aid. With the help of two well-trained nurses to pass syringes and prepare the next patient, before the previous one had finished, an average of 7 to 8 minutes was enough for each patient, including a brief questioning.

Each patient was reporting back in a week's time for his second injection, if required. From that moment and on, the clinic's patient turned to be his patient too, since his improvement lied in his hands. The non satisfying results demanded answers and each time the possible one should be searched among the following three: wrong diagnosis, wrong injected area or the injectors inadequacy. The answers were far from being easy. Trying to understand the reasons, he started to learn.

The idea behind infiltrations is similar to the notion of watering the plant in need instead of the field, which is the case when drugs are administered by mouth or the IM route. With local injections, the treated area receives adequate medication. The low absorption preparation of cortisone is consumed mainly locally and the amount that enters the general circulation is negligible and harmless. It is practically the treatment of choice for patients whose stomach, liver and kidneys, do not welcome drastic medications.

His postgraduate training in UK lasted five years. Apart of a short interval in general and vascular surgery, it concerned mainly orthopedics. Working under a variety of consultants, in totally five hospitals of England and Wales, he had to decide among different opinions. He gradually came to realize that he had to build his own beliefs, accepting or modifying the existing ones or adding new if he could.

The realization that spine was behind some orthopaedic problems, was built up gradually and a combined treatment started being tried on them later when back at home he had to face the Sudeck's syndrome cases which followed the Colley's fractures on patients already suffering of a cervical problem. When apart of the tender area, injections were also tried on the spine, the results were impressive. This treatment was applied successfully after this to any other Sudeck's syndrome since a spine history and local sensitivity was revealed to exist in all of them. Persisting postoperative pain in certain cases was found to be of this kind and not due to operative faults. Keeping on the lookout for similar conditions has led to the discovery of the facet syndromes described in this book.

Nikolaos Giantsios

REPRESENTATIVE FACET SYNDROME CASES

A ll syndromes displayed here, are those, which the author has verified and recognized himself as facet syndromes. As verification criterion was accepted the positive response to the local facet treatment. The involved in each syndrome specialties are mentioned under the titles.

Trigeminal Neuralgia (Neurology, Dentistry, Stomatology, ENT Surgery)

The identification of trigeminal neuralgia as a facet syndrome was accidental. This happened when one of the patients who was treated by him in the past for a brachial neuralgia, returned a few months later with this different kind of pain, which this time grew to an unsolved problem for those who had tried to help. The only sign connecting these two neuralgias were the same cervical facet joints, which were found again, tender on palpation. Although this kind of neuralgia was not of an orthopaedic surgeon's concern, the facet joints were. Trying his injections on them, the relief of pain was dramatic.

The dentist is quite often the one who is approached first by patients of this kind. It is the dental pain the one which drives them to him. The ENT surgeon might follow. Ear pain, dizziness and painful catarrh of the upper respiratory tract are possible manifestations. After these two specialists have tried and failed, then comes the neurologist to whose jurisdiction these cases belong to come with the right diagnosis. His treatment is some kind of heavy sedation. The stomatologist, when available, might be asked to help with the tongue causalgia, which frequently accompanies this condition. The average number of tablets these patients are taking daily might reach the 15 and when time comes to stop this treatment, they are advised to do it gradually, reducing the daily dose.

When these patients were questioned, about pain a couple of minutes after their neck was injected, their usual reaction was to bring up slowly their index finger and press the skin all over the face. The reply, which followed was that they could not touch it before. What they still felt were the needle pricks in their neck behind. What the surgeon had treated were cervical facet joints. The area where symptoms prevailed had no segmental relation to them. The same cervical facets were injected by him in the past for being responsible for the brachialgia or something else they had. This led him accept, that what he had treated this time was a different manifestation of the same facet syndrome.

A few examples might prove helpful. One of the early cases was a woman age 40, operator of a sewing machine. Her problem was pain, starting from the occiput, extending to the teeth in front one side, continuously day and night, over a period of three years.

She first addressed to a dentist who, finding a wide area of local tenderness, was persuaded that the problem was dental and started extracting one after the other the teeth of both jaws one side, trying to find the wrong one. With

19

her problem persisting, she was advised to visit an ENT surgeon who diagnosed sinusitis and suggested curettage. This did not help her either. A second ENT surgeon, agreeing with the diagnosis of his previous colleague tried the same, believing that his curettage would prove more effective. With her problem remaining, she addressed to a neurologist who after diagnosing a trigeminal neuralgia tried the best he could, having the same luck with the colleagues who had tried before.

The author was approached after this patient had heard of his injections. The palpation of the cervical spine revealed local tenderness on the suffering side. Realizing that he was dealing with an overuse syndrome, he felt that it was worth trying an injection on her. It was explained to the patient that her cervical spine was suspected to be the source of her problems and her job responsible for this. The only way to find out was to inject her neck. She was already prepared to accept this and proved so by saying "that's why I am here doctor". In her despair she would accept any treatment proposed to her. She was asked to return in a week's time if this first injection proved to be helpful.

She never showed up but reported back only eight months later praying for another injection when she felt an impending relapse of the pain. She was completely relieved from pain all this time through. Five years later, she was still symptoms-free when she escorted to his surgery her mother-in-law for a problem of hers. She was last seen twenty-five years later asking advice if she really needed treatment for osteoporosis. The cervical spine had never been a problem again. She had understood quite well her spine's limits to physical strain and that work was the one, which had to be changed and adjusted to her.

The undisputed fact in this case is that the patient found relief only after her cervical spine was injected. This left no room for doubt that spine was standing behind this trigeminal neuralgia. When at a later time the facet syndromes started being discussed, then in retrospect the author realized that what he had treated successfully was a cervical facet syndrome.

In regards to the dentist, the ENT surgeons and the neurologist, they obviously did not suspect that the cervical spine was behind the problem. They could not possibly know something for which nothing had been written till then. On what concerns the first two, the local vasomotor reactions within their territory had trapped them both. They both had a local problem; it was not just a referred pain. Whatever they touched was painful. None of them could say the problem is not mine.

The orthopedic surgeon was involved, when someone told this desperate patient that she had her headache cured by him. He was surprised to find out eight months later that a single facet infiltration had taken the pain away completely. He would not even know what he had cured if the patient had not mentioned the neurologist's diagnosis. He had the chance to verify that this entity is a facet syndrome handling successfully the same way the trigeminal neuralgias he had later come across.

A similar case is that of a female patient, age 65, whose complaint was a persisting brachial neuralgia. Over the previous few years she had all sorts of pain around the shoulder girdle and head. When she was questioned if she ever had any problems with her teeth, this came as a shock to her. She recalled that the previous year a different kind of pain had led to two teeth extractions and that the dentist, for whom she had been working as an assistant for over twenty years, confessed to her that both extracted teeth were healthy.

The author had not any hesitation to accept that her present neuralgia and the dental pain, which had led in the previous year to the teeth extractions, had both the same origin. He before had met this. This was actually the reason why this question was put on her.

The following third case is brought here in purpose of displaying the patient's difficulty to realize which specialty is the right one to handle his problem. This is the case of a woman around 70, a retired trained nurse, who had been repeatedly attended in the past for various musculoskeletal problems.

Once she appeared with a brachial neuralgia extending down the wrist accompanied by numbness of fingers. This followed a strenuous manual work and could not be correlated to any lesion of the cervical spine, which could possibly exert mechanical pressure on roots. The symptoms were attributed to a spasm of the vasa nervorum of the brachial plexus and the patient was relieved completely from pain and numbness after the tender cervical facets were injected. This was a straightforward case of a facet syndrome, easy to diagnose, since the suffering facets were correlated segmentally to the distribution of symptoms.

The same patient was seen a few months later with a completely different clinical picture, which started the day after entertaining friends. Trying to cut quinces to pieces for a special dish, pressing hard on both ends of the knife, she felt a snap in her neck. Severe pain to the left ear is how it started the day after. The pain soon spread to the eyes in front. Tongue causalgia, sore throat and burning sensation of nasal mucosa were added. It was only the tenth day, after the efforts of the involved specialists had failed, when the patient suspected that the cervical spine might be standing again behind her present problem and that she had to visit the orthopedic surgeon whose painful injections she really hated.

Injecting the tender facets solved her problem. The author's belief is that the facets he injected this time were the same with those he did a few months earlier to treat the brachial neuralgia. The clinical picture this time was completely different but the responsible facets the same. The explanation he could give was that this time different vasomotor centers were triggered and as rout of reaction was chosen the trigeminal nerve. The whole clinical picture was found compatible with a trigeminal neuralgia. This was actually what the preceded colleagues had diagnosed and were trying to treat.

On what concerns this clinical entity, the neurologists in general were never quite sure about its etiology. A virus involvement is often incriminated. The officially diagnosed as trigeminal neuralgia cases, the author happened to come across, proved to be facet syndromes. This diagnosis was his only option, since they responded only when the treatment was directed to the cervical facets.

Dysphagia (ENT Surgeons, Neurologists, Gastroenterologists)

The following case concerns a woman, around 50, who suddenly presented a serious swallowing problem. Her husband was searching in despair to find out which is the right specialty to deal with his wife's problem. The efforts of the involved doctors of three different specialties who were trying to help her along the last two months had failed. Her condition kept deteriorating.

Nikolaos Giantsios

The author was approached not for his medical services but to help them find the right doctor who could possibly help. He had treated this patient a couple of years earlier for a brachial neuralgia. He suggested seeing the patient first.

Finding the cervical facets again tender on palpation he thought worth trying an injection as he had done it in the past. This would at least give him time to think who might be the right specialist to refer her to. One week later, her husband rang to report that his wife was almost back to normal and prayed for a second injection. He could not stand living again the same agony watching his wife dying of starvation. For the following fifteen years this patient remained symptoms free. Three more dysphagia cases with sensitive cervical spine were treated this way with the same success.

Dysphagia is a problem, which does not concern an orthopedic surgeon. These few cases however, which sought his help, are an indication that some at least of the dysphagia cases could claim to be listed as facet syndromes.

One of these cases, an elderly man, around 70, returned six months after his swallowing problem was solved, with a facial palsy and pain of trigeminal distribution. There was numbness over his left cheek and upper lip, plus the typical facial paresis. That time it did not cross the author's mind that facial palsy, trigeminal neuralgia and dysphagia could be manifestations in sequence of the same facet syndrome. The truth is, that at that time he did not yet think in terms of facet syndromes the way he later did. It did not cross his mind to inject this patient's neck again. As he was later informed, the patient ended with perforation of his cheek.

Much later, on another case, the facial palsy was accompanied by tongue causalgia. Both of them responded to facet infiltration. They had to be accepted as different manifestations of the same facet syndrome.

Irritable Cough, Brachial Neuralgia, Cardiac Arrhythmia (Chest Specialists, Neurologists, Cardiologists)

A gynecologist addressed to the author for a brachial neuralgia he had, which had followed a persistent irritable cough. The patient, being a doctor himself, was led to suspect that some kind of obscure tumor in his lungs had now metastasized to the spine.

Injecting the tender facet joints the pain disappeared and so did the irritant cough. Both irritable cough and brachial neuralgia had to be accepted as manifestations in sequence of the same facet syndrome.

The same was the case with a female patient who was visiting physicians one after the other for an irritable cough over a period of three months. A brachial neuralgia was added on top of the chest problem. Reporting one week after receiving injection on her cervical spine, cough and neuralgia had both disappeared.

The same patient was seen on another occasion for a similar cervical problem. Cardiac arrhythmia was found on palpation. There was a pause after every three to four normal pulses. Mentioning this to her she protested by saying that the cardiologist, who had examined her recently had assured her that the cardiac function was checked to be perfect. The next day, after injecting her neck, both neuralgia and arrhythmia had subsided. The

25

Nikolaos Giantsios

explanation that both of them could well be manifestations of the same facet syndrome could not be denied.

The Cardiologists describe this arrhythmia as an extra-cardial one, a defense mechanism against external stimuli, which the heart is trying to avoid reacting this way and they are not worried much when coming across.

The mucosa of the upper respiratory tract is an area where peripheral vasomotor reactions can be caused by facet joints. Congestion of mucosa can affect drainage of sinuses, cause unexplained chronic inflammations, respiratory difficulties and so on. Sneezing attacks with rhinorrhoea were a frequent problem on a healthy young man who had to spend long hours working on his PC. The mechanical stress on his cervical spine was finally what the patient himself found out to be the cause. What he had noticed was that sneezing and rhinorrhoea started whenever he had to look upwards for more than a few minutes.

A few years ago the author was touring Syria with a group, mostly Americans. Sleep apnea was the problem for one of them. He had found solution with a CPAP device (Continuous Positive Airways Pressure). One day, while sitting in the hotel's internal garden in Damascus, one asked him to look upwards at the glass roof which decked the garden and watch the two men walking on it. He denied doing so explaining that this would make him feel dizzy.

Evidently his cervical facets had a problem, which was reacting whenever his spine was forced to hyperextension. What one would be allowed to wonder is if the cervical facets which were triggering dizziness when attempting to look upwards, were in some way involved with his sleep problem, a complete different clinical entity. Under different conditions the author would not resist the temptation to find out. One injection would probably give him the answer within the first couple of days.

Confusing Trans Specialties Symptomatology

One day the author runs into Ann, his children's English teacher. Her husband Bill had recently taken over the management of a private English School and started organizing everything electronically. The last few weeks he did not feel well. This worried her a lot. The doctors who attended him could not find any obvious reason, so they suggested admission to hospital for further investigation. The author offered to see him first.

The patient, a well-organized and hard working person, felt for the first time in his life, that something was going wrong. Dizziness and instability were what worried him most. He attributed the stiffness of his neck to the prolonged work he was doing lately on his PC.

Although his cervical spine was not particularly painful, it should be found out first if this was a part or the reason of his problem. This could be verified if he agreed to have his neck injected first. The patient, having heard of the author's injections, accepted it.

Three days later Bill rang to thank for getting back to normal. He asked explanations for how was it possible to think more clearly, to hear and see better, even colors to be brighter. It was obvious that the cervical facets were those, which were involved. By the moment they were treated all these functions were restored to normal.

A few years later the author run again into Bill's wife. She introduced him to her friend from London who had come to visit her. Turning to her she said "this is the doctor I was telling you about last night, the one who saved Bill six years ago with just one injection". This was an indirect feedback that things had happened this way.

It was a routine questioning on patients visiting him for problems related to their cervical spine, if further to the reason of their visit, they had any symptoms concerning vision and hearing. Some of them reported blurred vision, easy fatigue in reading, difficulty in focusing and occasional transient diplopia for which the ophthalmologist could not find an obvious reason. They usually reported on the next appointment that in addition to what they had come for, the ophthalmic or auditory symptoms had subsided.

Patients whose present problem was a facet syndrome mentioned unexplained fainting episodes in the past and urgent admissions to hospitals. Some of these patients had a history of retina detachment, after a trivial injury. A possible explanation which satisfied the author's suspicions was that the same facet joints he was treating that time, had triggered in the past a vasomotor reaction on the retina to the point a minimal trauma at a later stage to be enough to produce a fissure. Myopic persons are known to be prone to retina detachment. They are among those who exert more than anybody else mechanical stress on their cervical spine while trying to focus at work, even while wearing glasses. This might be a reason, why this may happen to them. This kind of simplified and arbitrary interpretations were the result of the author's lasting suspicion that eyes could not possibly be immune of facet interference since vision is an indispensable partner in the function of the locomotor system.

Acute Deafness (Personal Case Study: The Olive Tree)

The author had a personal experience with a problem concerning his hearing at the age of 75. He has an old olive tree in his garden that gives a lot of olives every year. Once, a few years ago, it took him three days to collect them one by one climbing on a ladder. He wondered for his stiff neck not protesting, been forced to work for two days in full extension. The third and last day, waking up after a short siesta, he realized that he was completely deaf from his left ear.

This reminded him of the farmers visiting him for a stiff neck, neuralgia, dizziness or ear noises after fruit collection or pruning of trees. This kind of work takes long hours using both arms while the cervical spine is forced to remain all along in full extension. Injections were those, which were helping them. This option was now not available for him at a moment he needed them. He did not know anyone of his colleagues to practice them on the cervical spine.

The ENT surgeon explained that he was seeing quite often cases of acute deafness. Some of them recover completely, some not. The etiology is not clear. A virus cause is often suspected. As far as treatment is concerned, some prescribe drugs which strive to keep the nerve cells alive providing better oxygenation, others heavy doses of cortisone. Since the local injections, which the author applied to others were not an option for him, he took both types of medication. Which means that his only choice was to water the field instead of the one plant in need. The amount of cortisone he took was many times more than that of the one injection and the amount that reached the facets one hundredth. His hearing recovered, by 30% only. The stereoscopic hearing was lost.

This example is clearly personal. The diagnosis of a facet syndrome is verified only by its positive response to a facet treatment. Local facet treatment in his case was not provided and consequently adequate confirmation is missing. This report might prove useful as a stimulus to those who might consider worth trying investigating if any of the acute deafness cases they come across are facet syndromes.

In the author's case, the ENT surgeon had to treat a suffering organ and save nerve cells from dying. If this case was a cervical facet syndrome, getting somebody to inject the facets would certainly help him do his job more effectively. By the moment the facets were properly attended, there would be no reason for them to perpetuate affecting the blood supply of the auditory nerve, if this was the mechanism of interference.

No doubt the ENT surgeons and Ophthalmologists are suspecting a central neurological involvement in some of their clinical entities. The question is how to verify what it really is and then how to treat it. The fact that the author himself has failed at a crucial moment for his hearing to verify the nature of his personal problem, this leads to the sad realization that the time when sufferers of these syndromes might start expecting this type of help, is not yet a matter of the near future.

Temporal Arteritis and Blindness

A female patient age 65 showed up one day with symptoms related to her cervical spine. She stated from the start that she was already on a treatment with steroids, five years now, for a temporal arteritis she was diagnosed to have and whatever treatment the author decided this should not interfere with the cortisone treatment she was already on. She was obviously concerned for the future of her eyes and appeared quite sure that the best treatment had been applied on her to prevent any damage on them.

The author felt that it would be a great mistake if anyone attempted to change this belief. Injecting her spine could have probably helped her present problem, but the threat of a serious future eye problem would remain a possibility. If so, the injections might be incriminated for any nasty outcome in future, so he avoided helping her. According to his beliefs the temporal arteries are potential facet's victims the same way eyes and auditory nerves are. Both temporal arteritis and blindness can appear as manifestations in sequence of the same facet syndrome but not as the consequence one of the other.

Instability and Dizziness

The ENT surgeons usually attend patients presenting these symptoms. Facet joints are reporting to the balance center and when suffering they might be the reason. Theoretically any one of them can cause these symptoms. In practice it was the cervical ones, which were found to prevail. It was not rare for instability to subside after injecting the lumbar spine only.

Chronic Headaches and Cervical Spine

A distinct group of lasting headaches has attracted quite early the author's interest. They were cases, which had resisted for years all sorts of therapies and responded to a single facet infiltration. Although found to start from the cervical facet joints, they could not be understood as facet syndromes the way the author understood them. Once they were successfully treated the result was permanent. They did not relapse. A history of trauma was traced for most of them. Whiplash injuries were later found to belong to this group and respond to this treatment.

The inability for quite long time to understand how a single facet infiltration could cure a headache, which had resisted all sorts of treatment for years, was what had triggered the author's curiosity to search for a satisfying answer. He was finally led to accept the possibility that the chiropractors knew, long before anybody else, how to treat these cases.

The manipulation of the cervical spine is the method they apply. Reading their descriptions on how they perform these manipulations, one is led to accept that this way they probably break adhesions, which happen to be there. Bending and rotating the spine to extreme positions is a maneuver, which succeeds to stretch them. This tension is transferred to pain sensors. This is the moment when the chiropractor, feeling his patient's discomfort, applies a carefully controlled jerk, which achieves to break them. Once this is done the pain disappears. What is not understood is why the chiropractors still keep the term "reduction" when referring to this process?

The muscular spasm, which immobilizes the cervical spine after an injury of a facet joint, is a protection mechanism against pain. This gives enough time for adhesions to form between the adjacent surfaces of an injured capsular fold. When this happens, any movement to unfold is resulting to pain. This is what happens after a whiplash injury. This will last for as long these adhesions remain there and will stop only after one will break them. This is what an expert chiropractor achieves.

Quite probably the same happens after injecting the spine. The basic difference with this kind of treatment is that the manipulation is not done by any chiropractor or doctor, but by the patient himself, when he, relieved from pain, tries instinctively to regain the lost range of movement by turning his head again and again to the direction he could not do before. It is the local anesthetic what permits this self-manipulation and cortisone the one which prevents new adhesions to form. Breaking adhesions is practically a new trauma. New ones may form again. Maybe this is the reason why the relief the chiropractor obtains is quite frequently temporary only. He cannot prevent the new ones to form again.

The following three cases, aim to contribute to this understanding. The first one concerns a woman aged 60 whose headache had never stopped through the last ten years. It was not recorded how it started. The pain went off completely and permanently after one facet infiltration only. There was no logic explanation how the injections had achieved it. What the author still recalls after injecting this patient's neck is to watch her turn her head to the stiff side again and again keeping saying, "Oh, I could not do this before." It took him many years to realize that what his patient was doing that moment in front of his eyes was the manipulation of her own spine. It was the local anesthetic the one which had allowed her to do this.

The second case is a narrated story by one of his patients. His headache started after a fall from his horse. It stopped suddenly seven years later after a second fall. Although this case was often recalled as a joke, the sensible answer was missing. A possible one matured much later. The second fall had just provided the manipulation, which the patient's neck desperately needed all these years to break the adhesions, which the first one had produced. Knocking his head against the ground provided the sudden jerk,

33

which the expert chiropractor would apply, if he had to treat this spine.

The third case concerns an agriculturist 39 years old who for the last 20 years was suffering of a continuous headache. He had finally accepted that he had to live with this pain for the rest of his life. It started at the age of 18 at a time when he suddenly realized that the time left for taking the admission exams to University was too short. Those two months of intensive studying were the hardest working period in his life. Injecting his cervical spine twenty years after his problem had started, one infiltration of facet joints was enough to free him from pain and keep it so for the following thirty years.

A trauma history is missing in this case. The way this had responded to treatment could be understood only in terms of adhesions involvement. The possibility that the prolonged mechanical strain had affected the articular capsule of a facet joint to reach the point for adhesions to form is beyond the author's experience to affirm. The lack of any other satisfying answer is what has led him accept this possibility.

According to this concept, adhesions within the facet joints attached to pain sensors of a capsular fold, is an acceptable explanation for these lasting headaches till a better one will appear to take its place.

Overuse Syndromes

These clinical conditions are the result of repeated mechanical strain on the muscle origins or their tendons. The mechanical factor is not questioned. Nevertheless it was observed that in certain of these cases, those who resisted to local treatment, the regional facet joints were found involved. This was attributed to the fact that the peripheral mechanical strain affects inevitably the spine too. When the latter is sensitized, it can enter the game. This concept was reached after the realization that insisting manifestations of these syndromes were responding favorably when the involved facet joints received attention.

Tennis Elbow

The medical term for this condition is *lateral epicondylitis of elbow* and as cause is accepted the repeated mechanical strain on the tendinous origin of the extensor muscles of wrist and fingers, most important for a firm grip. All functions done by the upper extremities are transferring mechanical stress to the cervical spine too. A repeated strain, which affects the elbow, can also affect the cervical spine.

Palpating the spine on certain of these patients, one detects tenderness of the cervical facets. Questioning these patients if further to their present problem have noticed any other symptoms, no matter if irrelevant, they often mention that they wake up in the morning with pain around the shoulders and occasionally instability with pins and needles down their legs. This was actually what had reported a woman, age fifty who came to the author's surgery with both elbows affected, worse on one side. She had at work to cut paper and occasionally cardboard with scissors all the day through, for the playing needs of the infants of her private nursery. She cried when told that she could not continue doing this any longer.

It is obvious that this kind of work was affecting her cervical spine too. The question of what had started the local inflammation, the direct repetitive stress to the elbow or the indirect one to the cervical facets, is not the subject of this discussion. The answer is that both are involved, since cases of this type are the difficult ones to treat and they respond when both elbow and spine are injected the same time. In other words, pronounced types of tennis elbow are responding well when treated as facet syndromes.

It was a routine process to check the cervical spine on each tennis elbow case and question the patient for any possible symptoms which could be relevant This questioning was helping the patients too to understand the nature of their problem and find out ways of modifying work habits. This patient, instead of having a second injection took as present a pair of electric scissors. The author in return, apart of the patient's gratitude, had one more case for his book.

LUMBAR FACETS & LOWER EXTREMITIES

The Upper Iliotibial Band Facet Syndrome, Piriformis Syndrome, Peritrochanteritis

The facets can trigger vasomotor inflammations at points of tendon insertions, round trochanters and structures of the deep fascia. The same is true for pes anserinus tendinitis, tender heel and plantar fasciitis. One can find by history and palpation affinity between them and lumbar facet joints.

The upper iliotibial band facet syndrome is a local vasomotor reaction of the upper part of this band at the insertion site of tensor fascia latae and the upper three quarters of the gluteus maximus muscle. This tenderness might extend downwards along the iliotibial band to the middle of the thigh and affect also the adjunctive fatty layer of the superficial fascia. It is a lumbar facet syndrome analogous to that of pes anserinus. The iliotibial band syndrome, which affects runners and bicyclists, is a completely different entity. It is an overuse syndrome due to friction of the lower part of this band over the lateral epicondyle of the femur before its insertion to the lateral tibial condyle.

37

At a deeper level, the insertions of gluteus maximus (the deeper fourth), gluteus medius, gluteus minimus and piriformis muscles on greater trochanter and the gluteal ridge might present a similar reaction. Peritrochanteritis is the term used to define this pain. Cases of these two groups have responded to a single infiltration when the involved facets were injected the same time. It may be the etiology of piriformis syndrome met on elderly people is the same. The way this condition was met when coming across, was that of a facet syndrome.

Pes Anserinus Syndrome and Aseptic Necrosis of the Medial Femoral Condyle

The term *"pes anserinus syndrome"* was first suggested by E.A.Nicoll to be used as a title for the type of pes anserinus tendinitis described in this book. This happened 25 years ago during one of his visits to Greece when the author had the chance to discuss with him his observation that the medial peri arthritis of knees, encountered mostly on women of heavy built and dilated superficial veins, was related to the lumbar spine. This was a clinical observation based on one hundred and thirty cases. They responded to treatment when both spine and knee problem were injected the same time.

E.A. Nicoll was the first consultant the author had worked for, while in UK, at the Royal Hospital in Chesterfield and at the time of this discussion he was honorary Publishing Editor of the Italian Orthopaedic Journal. He offered to publish a paper on this subject provided it was fully documented and he was assured that nothing had been written on this subject before.

The full documentation was out of question. Lab tests and X-Rs were not an important first step in private practice, especially when treating a purely clinical condition like this. Detailed data could not be provided. So the idea of publishing was abandoned but the suggested term "pes anserinus syndrome" was kept to appear first in this book 25 years later.

The muscular and joint strain is usually the cause when this condition is met on athletes. Apart of them, patients of older ages, especially women are those who often present this syndrome after moderate strain. This happens when the additional muscular and joint strain on knees happens at a time when the lumbar facet joints are already in trouble. This strain is affecting the spine too. The MRI finding, in cases dragging for long, is a disturbed endosteal circulation of the medial femoral condyle and the final outcome may be the bone necrosis.

Cases of this category on whom the facet treatment averted this ending are brought here to illustrate this. The first one concerns a woman, age 55, a fan of mountaineering, who was finally told by the surgeon who was treating her, that her knee problem in spite of all the treatment she had, would probably end as an aseptic necrosis of the medial femoral condyle.

The MRI had reported evidence of impairment of the intraosseous blood supply. Her case was diagnosed to be an impending aseptic necrosis and was submitted to some sort of expensive treatment, which lasted for seven to eight weeks. The treatment was aiming to save the bone cells by providing better oxygenation. The new MRI, eight weeks later did not change the picture. The pain persisted the same and now the other knee had started bothering her too. Her doctor's belief was that the bone necrosis was most probably established in the knee, which was affected first.

Panic was what drove the patient to seek a second opinion. The diagnosis was that this case was from the start a pes anserinus syndrome and not a knee joint arthritis. Spine and tendon area were both found tender on palpation. The patient remembered that a low back pain had put her in bed a few weeks before her knees started hurting. It was explained to the patient that she could possibly be helped if she accepted, apart of the tender area over the pes anserinus tendon, to have her spine injected too, although this area was not a pressing problem for her at the time. The belief was that the lumbar spine was the source of the knee problem.

After two weekly sessions of spine and knee injections, the pain subsided. The MRI, done the third week, showed complete restoration of the intraosseous circulation of the medial femoral condyle back to normal. Although the author has treated hundreds of these cases, he cannot provide information on how frequently this MRI finding accompanies these cases. He did not consider that a test of this kind could prove of any diagnostic value for a purely extra articular condition like this. The only MRIs he has seen concerning this clinical entity were those, the patients had already done earlier before coming to him.

In retrospect this knee test, although ignored by him initially as meaningless, proved most helpful to reveal an underlying intraosseous vascular threat on patients whose spine had remained without a proper treatment for long.

A second similar case concerns a woman around 60, with a history of 1st degree spondylolisthesis at the L4-L5 level and a persisting knee pain. She had to go up and down stairs a lot of times daily. The MRI reported an upset of the intraosseous vascular supply to the medial femoral condyle and the threat of an impending aseptic necrosis. Been told by her doctor that the bone necrosis was a possibility, which could hardly be stopped, the patient was desperately running for other opinions.

The diagnosis was that this case was again a pes anserinus syndrome from the start. Full clinical recovery and restoration of the MRI picture to normal were obtained after two weekly sessions of treatment, injecting both knee and lumbar facets. After that the patient knew that apart of avoiding stairs, the spine was the one she had to take care of for the rest of her life if she wished to keep her knees safe.

In both examples the patient's problem was finally considered to be a facet syndrome from the start and was treated as such. Both spine and knees were injected. The congestion of the femoral condyles subsided in both cases. Treating hundreds of knees this way none of them ended to bone necrosis. The author's belief is that what is known as "idiopathic necrosis of the medial femoral condyle", is nothing else than the end result of a pes anserinus syndrome, which failed to be diagnosed and treated as such. The story of what happens with the upper end of the same bone is not much different. This is a subject, which will never stop demanding a satisfactory answer. A similar approach concerning the hip joint is presented later in this book.

Swollen ankles are certainly an aesthetic problem for women. This edema is present as a symptom in many of the pes anserinus cases. It subsides impressively the next couple of days after spine and knees have been injected.

The pes anserinus tendinitis can exist without any facet involvement. If one has to climb stairs, especially circular and narrow with steps of 20cm or higher, he/she can easily get a pes anserinus tendinitis. This can subside with rest and avoiding stairs, with or without medication. The vasomotor manifestations locally and in the vicinity, and the persistence of pain in spite of rest and use of non-steroids, are what make the difference between a simple tendinitis and the syndrome.

The pes anserinus syndrome may coexist with knee OA and should be treated before proceeding to a total knee replacement. The failure to realize this coexistence can lead to a persisting postoperative pain after an otherwise successful knee operation.

Plantar Fasciitis and Tender Heel

Plantar fasciitis and tender heel are accepted to be manifestations of a facet syndrome with the lumbar facets to stand behind. The combined spine and local treatment is what has proved to be effective on them.

Facets & Segments; the Paradox

Considering that online communication exists between facet joints and all systems collaborating with the balance center, the proprioceptors of any one of these joints, no matter how remote they are, have theoretically equal chances of access to vasomotor centers of any one of these systems and trigger them when in trouble. The afferent channels, which these distress signals follow, are the communication routes from facets to centrum along the spinal cord. When these centers react the efferent channels are those, which each one of these systems is using. The segmental related to facets roots are usually ignored. This fact is rendering every facet syndrome to behave more or less as a paradox.

This was realized first when treating patients with symptoms concerning both lumbar and cervical areas. The examples that follow are aiming to illustrate the diversity of clinical pictures, which each time these syndromes might present.

One of the cases which first drew attention to this fact concerns a woman, age 55, who showed up with all sorts of pain round the shoulder and pelvic girdles, radiating down to arms and legs. She had her daughter's wedding in three weeks' time and was desperate for help. She had been helped in the past with injections on her lumbar spine for pain radiating down the legs. It was explained to her that this time, the wide distribution of pain did not permit both areas to be injected the same time. She had to decide where to start. Having on this first appointment her lumbar spine injected only, she returned one week later to report that the pain from the cervical area had completely gone.

The minimal amount of the low absorption cortisone, which might have entered the general circulation, could not justify this dramatic effect on the cervical area. Similar medication by mouth had already been tried on her and failed. Segmental relation of lumbar facets with the cervical area does not exist. What was left to be gathered was that proprioceptors from lumbar facets had attacked vasomotor centers of both pelvic and shoulder girdles. After this, when coming across similar cases, the suggestion was to treat the lumbar spine first.

This paradox of having cervical problems improved after injecting lumbar facets only was repeated in quite a number of cases. On all of them it was the lumbar spine the one which was re-injected if symptoms related to this area still demanded help.

This was found to happen also the other way round. The problem of an elderly woman was an acute cervical pain, which appeared after trying to hang for drying a heavy blanket. She had in mind to come before this had happened, for an injection to her lumbar spine, because her legs could no longer keep up with her when going out for shopping. Injections to this area had worked on her successfully, a couple of times in the past. This time the injection she had to her neck helped her legs too. Calling to report that the cervical pain had gone she stated that her legs improved also and did no longer need help for the time being.

This paradox, of pain being relieved in areas which had no segmental relationship to the injected facets, was the reason of distrust towards the drug companies who claimed that the action of their low absorption cortisone product was consumed mainly locally with minimal and negligible entrance to the general circulation. This distrust lasted till the time it was realized that treated remote facets were those which brought the improvement and not any absorbed cortisone from the injected area.

A relevant paradox is the following case. It concerns a male patient age 50 with a persisting pain in one of his knees. This was diagnosed to be a pes anserinus tendinitis and was treated as a lumbar facet syndrome by injecting both spine and knee area. The paradox with this case was that this patient kept his next appointment just to satisfy his curiosity. His other problem over the same period was a persisting headache, which his neurologist had failed to find out what was causing it. Realizing that the headache went off together with the knee pain he wondered if the knee was responsible for the headache he had.

That time this was met by the author as an irrelevant coincidence and was often recalled as a joke. Obviously his experience at that time was not the needed one to let him accept that the lumbar proprioceptors, which had caused the knee problem, were responsible for his headache too. By the moment the lumbar facets were treated, knee pain and headache went off. What cannot be excluded is the involvement of proprioceptors of the pes anserinus area, which entered the game following those of the spine. Suffering proprioceptors of tendons or peripheral joints have theoretically equal chances of access to vasomotor centers of systems collaborating with the balance center and trigger them with result organs controlled by them to be affected.

A female patient age 75 approached the author four months after the drilling operation she had for an osteochondral defect in one of her knees, had failed to relieve her from pain. The bone necrosis appeared six months after the knee pain had started. The original diagnosis was knee arthritis, which resisted all sorts of treatment and ended with an osteochondral defect. There was a history of low back pain on and off along the last two years.

On examination, a knee effusion was present. On palpation both pes anserinus area and lumbar spine were found tender. It was considered that this case was from the start a pes anserinus syndrome which not having received a facet treatment, had led to the osteochondral defect.

Both facets and pes anserinus area were infiltrated. The joint was aspirated and injected with cortisone to provide relief to the intra articular problem and to calm down the joint capsule proprioceptors which were probably also upset.

The patient was visiting the same period an Ophthalmologist once a month for an eye problem she had the same period. Coming from another town she asked if her next appointment could be arranged in a month's time to coincide with the one she had with the eye specialist.

Nikolaos Giantsios

On her second appointment the knee's condition was found much improved and the elicited information on what concerned the eye was that it's condition was found to be stabilized. On her third appointment it was decided that knee and spine did no longer need any further treatment. On what concerned the eye, the information was that the ophthalmologist, impressed by an unexpected improvement, decided to stop his monthly injections to the eye and just monitor it.

The orthopedic surgeon did not exclude from the start the possibility that both knee and eye problem were manifestations of the same facet syndrome. In other words the autonomic nervous system, responding to repeated distress signals from lumbar proprioceptors, attacked both knee and eye, the same time or in sequence. The synchronous improvement of knee and eye after treating suffering lumbar proprioceptors, allowed himself to entertain the idea that his injections had by coincidence helped the ophthalmologist to save the eye. The eye problem concerned the macula.

The eye's condition one year later remained steady. The ophthalmologist was happy to see his patient helped by him and considered this lasting improvement compatible with a regression stage not uncommon for this kind of disease. On what concerned the knee the patient was warned by the orthopaedic surgeon that the only way to keep it safe was taking care of her spine.

Evidently this kind of approach could not be shared with any ophthalmologist, even with the one who was treating this patient. The orthopaedic surgeon could not provide any convincing evidence that both of them were treating a different manifestation of the same disease. The fact that the eye improved markedly after the responsible lumbar facets were injected could hardly be accepted by any one to be anything more than a simple coincidence.

Unexplained positive results met on similar incidents were what was feeding the author's suspicions that facet joints could well stand behind eye problems. Perceptible evidence is not the kind of information, which the ANS is willing to provide. Nevertheless this system is eager to provide answers when asked and these are the positive or negative response when treatment is tried on facet joints.

Treating these syndromes is similar to playing a game planned for two. The ANS is the other player acting on behalf of the patient. He is the one who puts the rules and can change them each time. He stands by watching, ready to grand success to the one who will try. In this paradox game there is no winner and loser. Both players stand on the same side, one of them injecting and the other watching. The result will either satisfy or disappoint them both. The winner or loser is the patient.

Evidently, only the specialists involved, if they will ever decide to investigate this field can officially verify cases of this kind as facet syndromes. The proof they might get can be statistical only. If the ophthalmologists will ever decide to do this, they will certainly need a spine surgeon to help them with the spine approach. If they will not, they will never find out. Then cases like this, will certainly have a place as science fiction stories and will remain as stimulus only for the occasional naive artist who might come again across. The most he will get is the satisfaction of a new discovery. This will hardly touch the rest.

No need to say that all cases displayed in this chapter had strictly followed the same rules, which every facet syndrome does. The sense of paradox mentioned in the title existed only in the author's mind. This was happening to him quite often in early times whenever coming across conditions he could hardly understand.

Sudeck's Syndrome

Sudeck's syndrome (Reflex Sympathetic Dystrophy Syndrome - RSDS) is a complication, which affects almost 5% of minor trauma or surgery on the upper and lower extremities. It is a most painful and incapacitating condition, some sort of a non-septic local inflammation, affecting mainly the small joints of the extremities. Its social and financial cost is enormous. The autonomous system is incriminated of being involved and surgeons have a really hard time trying to cope with its treatment.

The author, being preoccupied with the idea that persisting peripheral post-traumatic pain could be related to existing spine problems, started injecting the spine when there was evidence that the latter was involved. The feeling was that trauma or surgery had come in a moment when spine had already its own problems and it was spine the one who triggered and maintained this complication. Treating both spine and peripheral problem, proved to be most effective. When he finally realized that what he was treating all these years was nothing else than suffering facet joints, this led him accept that Sudeck's osteodystrophy was nothing else than a further clinical picture caused by them.

The local problem in this clinical entity cannot be treated effectively as long as the suffering facet joints are ignored. The local vasomotor reaction is severe and requires meticulous infiltration of every single affected small joint.

Persisting pain after treating a Colles' fracture in elderly ladies with cervical problems was quite a frequency. It was irrelevant to how good the reduction and immobilization was. Quite often these patients were complaining for pain going up and down the arm and their most frequent complaint was that the cast was too heavy for them. By the time the cast was removed it revealed a painful oedema, which was foretelling a difficult recovery.

All these restless patients were considered candidates for this complication and were warned in time for the difficulties, which might follow by the time the cast was removed. If considerable pain persisted slowing down the mobilization then local and spine infiltration might be needed. Physiotherapy could help them only after the painful oedema had subsided. The change to a lighter acrylic cast proved helpful for them when done by the end of the 2nd week after reduction. Informing these patients before hand for things that might follow, prepared them accept whatever treatment was suggested to them on the way to recovery. This way, the typical Sudeck's atrophy picture was always prevented.

Sudeck's syndromes were always a welcome challenge to treat. A desperate male patient around 60 appeared one day with a swollen and bluish foot. He could not endure even the pressure of the bed sheet on it. His problem started eight months earlier after a sprain of his forefoot during the move to another town. This happened at a time when his lumbar spine had its own problems. The recent X-R films he had brought with showed an almost complete demineralization of tarsal and metatarsal bones. The efforts of the previous colleagues who had tried all treatments available had failed and the patient himself was terrified with the idea of losing his leg.

It was explained to the patient that a treatment with local injections would be tried. At the same time the spine should be injected too, because it was believed that this was the one, which had turned a minor injury to a major

49

problem. This treatment would be repeated in a week's time if this first one turned to be helpful. He reported back and had four totally weekly sessions of local infiltrations. The lumbar spine was injected twice only. Edema and pain subsided quickly. It took two weeks for the patient to attempt partial weight bearing. By the fifth week the physiotherapist took over. In three months the x-rays showed that the restoration of bone density was on the way.

Quite a number of these syndromes were successfully treated this way. The frozen shoulder is accepted to be the end result of a non-treated Sudeck's syndrome where a persisting joint synovitis triggered by upset cervical facet joints has led to extensive adhesions between inflamed surfaces of capsular folds. Vanishing bone is probably a similar entity.

Injecting the facets only, one cannot cure a Sudeck's syndrome. Any peripheral inflammation should be thoroughly infiltrated. Soft tissue therapists cannot offer help to these patients unless joint and spine problems have received promptly the proper medical attention before been sent to them.

Hip Osteoarthritis and Loosening of Implants

Although the total hip replacements were one of the author's favorite objects, it took him too long to realize that hip OA is nothing else than the end result of a lumbar facet syndrome.

What he had realized earlier was that most of the hip OA cases he had dealt with had a spine problem too and that the hip replacements he had performed on them, had a longer lifetime when this coexisting spine problem was properly looked after all the way along the postoperative time.

Inflow evidence along practicing hip surgery in over two hundred cases, was pointing the lumbar facets to play a role in loosening of implants. This belief was gradually reached when the author realized that his hip arthroplasties were lasting much longer than the average. The only extra care these patients had received was the close follow up of their spine problem all the way along the postoperative years. This led him assume that possibly his injections were those who prevented the facets to demolish what he had earlier built in. The realization that the same facet joints were those who had destroyed the hip at the first place, followed much later. An attempt to display this concept according to which facet joints are those who stand behind the etiology of both hip OA and loosening of implants are the two case studies, picked up among a lot of similar, starting from the end of events.

Case Study I (Lasting of Implants)

This first case which displays the facet's attitude toward implants, concerns a woman who at the age of 55 had a cemented metal to metal McKee-Farrar prosthesis on one side and four years later a plastic to metal on the other hip, cemented too.

Living in another town she was attended when needed by the local colleagues. She was returning back each time she was told that one or the other hip required revision. What each time was diagnosed was that the problem concerned the spine and points of muscular insertions in the vicinity of the operated hip. The treatment this patient was each time receiving were the paravertebral injections for the facets and the infiltration of any local tenderness of tendon insertions round the hip with cortisone and local anesthetic. The patient was each time reassured that the problem concerned the spine, not the hips. It was the spine she should be taking care of if she wished her hips to last. This went on and off for the next thirty years.

Thirty-seven years after the first hip replacement this patient underwent revision surgery. It was because of the failure of the implant, which sustained a fatigue fracture at the level the ball was melded to the stem. The surgeon who performed the revision was kind enough to send the removed implants back to his colleague who had implanted them 37 years ago, plus to provide the information that the other hip he had implanted 4 years later was still clinically sound.

The author's experience is limited to a number not exceeding much the two hundred hip replacements. Most of the early cases were cemented and revisions on them were limited to a relatively small number, may be less than 10%. Later on, when stems improved in shape, his interest grew in favor of the non-cemented. Their number is much smaller. He cannot recall revising any one of them. Almost all cases had received spine injections when needed along the years that followed the operation. The average time of implant lasting cannot be estimated since most of these patients had taken the implants away when dying.

What one can infer from this example is that quite early the surgeon suspected the spine to be a potential danger for his operations. The good fitting alone, although important, could not be the reason why his arthroplasties lasted much longer than the average. The importance of medullary reaming lies on the fact that it ensures the immobilization the bone cells need the first postoperative period to stabilize the implants by building new bone round them. It brings the implant in contact to solid bone and increases the contact surface leaving smaller gaps for the osteoblasts to fill. Bone is a living organ with osteoblasts, which will repair any microscopic fractures, which might happen at the contact area after stress or minor injury.

When the facet joints are in trouble, their proprioceptors can upset the normal blood supply to the bone that hosts the implants and prevent the bone cells from repairing a possible damage. They achieve this hazard through the vasomotor centers of the musculoskeletal system to which they have access.

In effect, the role of the surgeon who all these years periodically injected the spine was the protection of the bone cells by keeping the facet proprioceptors calm. Tender areas round the greater trochanter and iliotibial band are points of insertion of the gluteal muscles, piriformis and of tensor fasciae latae. This tendinitis is considered to be a local vasomotor reaction triggered by the facets. Now the tendon proprioceptors have entered the game too. The infiltration of these points is equally important with those of the facet joints. In other words a successful hip operation is only the start of a long journey. Any problem met all the way along, triggered by the facets, should be dealt with effectively if one wishes the implants to serve these patients all the life through.

The author had achieved his patients' cooperation for this close follow up, by injecting their spine before hip surgery. This was necessary to let them understand which pain surgery would relieve them from. This way they understood that their problem was a dual one and that their spine should be watched closely afterwards. This follow-up was offered free of charge to hesitant patients to protect them from suspicion that exploitation might be standing behind.

Nikolaos Giantsios

Case study II (Etiology of Hip OA)

This case refers to the start of events, the etiology of hip OA. It concerns a civil engineer, who at the age of 27 was first seen with a low back pain attributed to intense office work, technical drawing in particular. One paravertebral injection every three years on average, was enough to keep him fit along the following thirty years when the usual non-steroids did not help. There was no X-R evidence of any disc or other spine lesion through all these years.

At the age of 50 he was involved in a car accident resulting to a horizontal linear fracture of the Rt. acetabular fossa. The weight bearing part of the joint, according to diagnostic methods of that time, appeared to be intact. His hip did well just keeping off weight bearing for three months. The feeling of a pull at the front of the joint when opening his pace was the only symptom left. This was attributed to adhesions between psoas tendon and the hip capsule. The clinical estimation was that this hip did not deserve to end as an arthritic one. Seventeen years after the accident, the injured hip started hurting. At the same time the patient presented micturition problems.

The orthopaedic surgeon who was treating him that time diagnosed posttraumatic hip arthritis for which treatment without surgery should not be expected. With the pain increasing the patient had to use crutches for a period of three months. He was told that the solution would finally be the total joint replacement. The micturition problem, which started as a difficulty to start urination and a diminished flow, was evolving to almost incontinence. At this stage the urologist unable to help came to conclude that he was dealing with a neurogenic bladder and suggested that the patient should better see the surgeon who was taking care of his spine in the past.

This is how the patient returned to the author seven months after the start of the present problems. The patient was limping with pain. The internal rotation of the hip was restricted and painful. The ordinary X-R films were within normal on what concerned the joint space. Small osteophytes were traced at the acetabular rim. The MRI reported an upset of the blood supply both to femoral head and acetabulum, an intra-osseous marrow edema in particular. All evidence was pointing to an early stage of hip OA. The patient admitted that he had neglected his spine lately, considering its deterioration as a natural evolution of the aging process.

The impression was that the periodic low back pain of the past had now evolved to a new stage where hip arthritis and bladder problem had entered as different manifestations of the same facet syndrome. This had to be proved. The patient was told that his neglected spine should be treated first. This would possibly lead to the understanding of the hip problem. The latter would be dealt with afterwards. On this first appointment the tender lumbar facets were injected plus the tender psoas tendon in front of the joint. The hip joint itself was not touched. This was not a scientific decision but a defense measure to protect his injections from taking the blame for any nasty future outcome. After this case there was no hesitation to inject straight away any suffering hip joint considered to be Hip OA at the start.

The patient returned one week later to report that he did no longer need the crutches. Even the bladder problem started to improve. This was the best response the surgeon could expect. It confirmed his initial suspicion and pointed clearly the treatment he had to follow. Being preoccupied with the belief that the idiopathic necrosis of the medial femoral condyle is the end result of a neglected lumbar facet syndrome, this case was the proof he was waiting for to find out if what happens to the upper end of this bone is not much different.

At this second appointment, in addition to the facets and psoas, the joint was injected too. This, apart of relieving the joint, would cover the possibility that proprioceptors of the joint capsule were upset too. In such a case they might continue protesting, perpetuating the problem. This was the only intra-articular injection this patient has received. Two more weekly sessions followed injecting facets and psoas tendon, infiltrating also the anterior hip joint capsule where adhesions with the psoas tendon were suspected to exist since the time of the hip injury 17 years ago. The MRI, done three weeks after the start of the injection treatment reported marked improvement of the blood supply to both femoral head and acetabulum. The last MRI, two weeks later, reported full restoration of the intraosseous circulation to normal.

The Urologist was happy with his diagnosis seeing his patient cured. He now knows that this neurogenic bladder case was a lumbar facet syndrome. This discovery was all accidental. It was actually the side effect of a treatment meant to help the hip. This was the surgeon's main concern. It is for the Urologists now to decide which of their neurogenic bladder cases are possibly facet syndromes. The one under discussion was related to the L5-S1 facet joints.

On what concerns the hip joint, things are not so easy to analyze. There is a history of injury seventeen years ago. After such a long time one can hardly accept this arthritis as a post traumatic one. It was not only the facets, which were injected. The psoas muscle and tendon, the anterior joint capsule and once the joint itself were injected although the intra articular injections cannot treat a hip OA.

The interpretation, which was built up gradually was that spine was the source of the problem and that the rest, joint arthritis, psoas tendinitis, and intra osseous arteritis, were all secondary vasomotor reactions triggered by the spine. In other words, quite early, the hip OA was accepted as a dual problem and with the years passing, spine to be the one who had started it. This case was the milestone which turned the author's suspicions to a firm belief that

> "... Hip OA is just the end result of a non-treated lumbar facet syndrome."

He started recalling cases from the past, seen at the early stage of the disease, which had also responded to this way of treatment. These cases had really puzzled him. He was led to consider them as his diagnostic failures, since, according to what is generally accepted, what he had cured could not possibly be hip OA since the course of events in this disease entity cannot be reversed. He cannot forget his embarrassment when in a reunion meeting one of his old school mates thanked him publicly for having saved his hip twenty years earlier. He was one of these cases the author was still in doubt. Even at that time, thirty years after the start of his career he was not yet ready to accept that the answer to the etiology issue of hip OA could be a simple one.

The spine in this case had to be re-injected a few times during the next four years. It was evident that only an intervertebral fusion could possibly help to stop the spine problem. All this time the patient was convinced that the hip problem did no longer exist and the author was led to believe that even seven months after the start, this disease is still reversible. The hip pain relapsed four years later when the spine deteriorated again and at that time the patient decided instead of injections to give to his spine a chance trying a course of acupuncture. The hip condition kept deteriorating and the joint space presented the typical narrowing. Evidently the persisting spine problem remained a continuous threat for the joint.

At this stage the patient decided to have his spine fused. This done, relieved him from the spine pain but his hip could not longer be helped. Could the hip be saved if the spine fusion had been done earlier? This is a question done in retrospect. The patient himself was convinced at that time that hip problem did no longer exist and the surgeon had not any convincing excuse to push his patient to do the spine fusion earlier. Hip surgery followed soon after. This has helped the spine fusion to last.

This case, apart of revealing an interaction between spine and hip, can hardly convince anybody else apart of the author that hip OA is the result of a lumbar facet syndrome and as such a preventable disease.

Treating the hip OA as a facet syndrome at its start, the surgeon is bound to be a loser. Apart of his own satisfaction and his patient's gratitude, he will never have the evidence required to prove his achievement. He cannot convince anybody. The label of this disease is the bone necrosis and the narrowing of the joint space. When one prevents them from appearing the evidence of what one has cured is missing. This brings up the importance of involvement of more than one surgeon in any future research on this subject. They will have to decide in common for the identity of the sample cases relying on clinical criteria only since these should be cases of an early stage when irreversible bone changes have not appeared yet. It is self-understood that only surgeons, well experienced on this kind of treatment, can obtain reliable results.

In conclusion, according to this concept, Hip OA and loosening of implants are manifestations in sequence of the same facet syndrome. From the moment a healthy hip is selected as the target of a facet's protest, no matter if treated successfully on the start, it will never stop depending on facets' mercy. The same is valid for implants if they have to follow. Taming the spine is the only way this disease can be met.

Sinking Hips

One of the bilateral hip arthroplasties the author had performed, was a female patient age 60 who had an L4-L5, 1st degree spondylolisthesis too. She had heavy family obligations and had to report back quite frequently with low back pain and tenderness at points of muscle insertions round the hips. She was responding to the paravertebral injections and to local infiltrations of tender spots. She finally developed bilateral sinking arthroplasties.

This case is one of those recalled from the past. The author cannot be certain if this case was hip OA or sinking hips from the start. What is certain is that a spine problem existed. Sinking hips is another clinical entity of obscure etiology. It will be no surprise if facet joints will finally be found to stand behind. If such is the case, spine should be the one, which should be treated first before dealing with the suffering hips.

Facets & Late Sciatica

It is not rare for someone, who had a successfully operated PID in the past to report back some years later with sciatica and intermittent claudication, on the same or the contralateral side. The Lasegue's sign is usually negative. What the MRI usually reports, is the narrowing of one or more of disc spaces and the bulging of a couple of discs. Once the SLR reaches the 90 degrees, it makes no sense talking about pressure on any nerve root. The sciatica in these cases can well be due to a spasm of the vasa nervorum triggered by the worn out facet joints which were led to this condition having to work in subluxation after the approximation of the vertebral bodies.

These cases usually respond when the involved facet joints are injected. There is a tendency for pain to recur whenever these patients exceed their limits. The same is true for PID cases of the past, which have responded to conservative treatment. When cases of these two groups are led to theater for decompression, the failure rate is usually high. It is the stabilization of spine what they really need. It is the intervertebral fusion the one which provides immobilization to the suffering facets.

The author's belief is that the whole talk about unstable spine does not concern the disc space but the facet joints themselves. These facets can be the cause of any kind of sciatica even a severe one which can lead to a drop foot. A bulging disc is quite often a part only of the problem. It is the spasm of vasa nervorum the one which aggravates it. This can be verified injecting the spine before leading the patient urgently to theater.

Low back pain, muscular pelvic pain and peritrochanteric pain are recurrent problems. The PVI might be enough for the first two. The peritrochanteric pain is a vasomotor reaction at points of muscle insertions and apart of the facet infiltration, the local one is equally important.

Having the experience of both operative and conservative treatment, surgeons can decide which one is best for the patient. Starting with injections one comes gradually to realize that a lot of these cases can do well without surgery. Many of the sciatic cases have nothing to do with root pressure. They are simply cases where the lumbar facets have triggered a spasm on the vasa-nervorum. When this problem cannot be met with conservative measures then the spinal fusion is what remains to be considered.

Spastic Paraparesis

The purpose of this chapter is to provide evidence that certain at least of the spastic paraparesis cases, should be recognized as facet syndromes. This concept was originally based on a case, which for a period of eight years was repeatedly diagnosed and treated ineffectively by more than one neurologist as a hereditary spastic paraparesis. The spasticity subsided only after the involved lumbar facets were injected.

Spastic paraparesis is the clinical condition, which appears when messages starting from the upper motor neurons are partially blocked on their way down along the corticospinal tract. The receivers of these messages are the lower motor neurons, which control the muscles of the lower extremities. When this happens the result is the spastic gait. When the blocking of messages is complete, the result is the spastic paraplegia. These two entities have been described as "Hereditary Spastic Paraparesis" and "Hereditary Spastic Paraplegia" respectively, the second being usually the ending of the first. It was Adolph Strumpell the one who first described these two entities in 1883, as a heterogeneous group of a hereditary character.

The case study, which follows, belongs to this group. On what concerns the etiology, this case was found by the author to be related to the lumbar facet joints. As far as he knows, spastic paraparesis has not yet been described as a facet syndrome. His belief is that this specific case is. The importance of this realization lies on the fact that facet syndromes can be   successfully treated.

The following case was diagnosed and treated over a period of eight years as a Hereditary Spastic Paraparesis, the only available label for this clinical entity up to now. It concerns a male patient age 70, a chemist and inventor, who at the age of sixty sold his successful business in the field of applied chemistry to become a vine grower and wine producer. This hobby, which soon turned to be his new job, challenged him for harder physical involvement. Being himself an extremely fit man, he did not mind working harder.

At the age of 62 he presented the spastic gait. This resisted all sorts of therapies. Physiotherapy was getting him worse. Cortisone by mouth provided only temporary relief. He hated the spasmolytic and sedative drugs for degrading his vitality without any result in gait. There were short intervals of unexplained improvement when he could walk freely. These could not be correlated with any treatment and did not last more than a few hours, maximum a day. The patient having enjoyed intervals of improved gait had a strong belief that his invalidity could not be a permanent one. He never gave up hoping and seeking for a better answer.

The periodic intervals of unexplained improvement, mentioned by the patient, was what had triggered the author's interest when he was approached. This excluded a permanent lesion of the upper motor neurons. What could be considered as a possibility, was a periodic interference on their function. The nerve tissue is most sensitive to changes in its blood supply. The motor neurons themselves could not survive repeated ischemic episodes. Their long fibers, the axons, could possibly do. If one is ready to accept the vascular interference, this should be searched somewhere along the corticospinal tract, where the long fibers of the upper motor neurons are descending to meet the lower motor neurons.

The lower lumbar facet joints were found tender on palpation. The patient admitted periodic attacks of low back pain, which occasionally were severe. This information raised the suspicion of a remote possibility that lumbar facets were those who triggered the vascular problem along the corticospinal tract. The facet's involvement in this case could be verified only after finding and injecting them. The patient agreed to have his lumbar spine injected and to return in a week's time to report the result. At this first contact the L4-L5 and L5-S1 facets were infiltrated on both sides with cortisone and local anesthetic.

On his second appointment, one week later, the patient appeared convinced that the right treatment was found at last and on his third appointment, four weeks after the start of this treatment, he stated that this period was the longest relief of spasticity he ever had along the eight years of his suffering. He expressed this belief by stating that now he could control his legs when approaching a door and did not have to use both hands to stop him of falling against. He was anxious to restart his long daily walking.

Considering that the treatment, which has changed this patient's life, concerned the facets joints only, the diagnosis of a facet syndrome was left to be the only option. It revealed where the triggering factor was born. Although the patient was happy being able to walk freely, the swaying gait did not recover. Some of the axons of the upper motor neurons had obviously been destroyed along these eight years. What could not be estimated was the degree of damage already inflicted to the nutrient blood vessels along the corticospinal tract.

The belief is that the blood vessels were what the vasomotor center had attacked. The triangle of interaction in facet syndromes is between the facet joints where the stimulus is born, a vasomotor-center, which is triggered to react and the vascular supply to a nerve or organ where the vasomotor reaction appears. What has happened to the axons was the consequence of the vascular damage.

A few weeks later the patient returned with a relapse. He had just tried to accelerate his recovery by adding spine exercises and taking a five hours tour inspecting his neglected vineyard. It was too early for his spine to stand a test of this kind. Furthermore the crippled vascular supply to the corticospinal tract could not cope with the patient's wish for a return to normality. Unfortunately this treatment had reached the patient too late to reverse the neurologic damage. What it succeeded was to release the spasm and possibly prevent any further destruction of the long axons of the upper motor neurons. These neurons had lost control on a considerable number of the lower motor neurons. He had from now and on to rely only on what had been left and try to increase the muscular strength if possible. The release of spasticity remained steady along the months that followed. The spine was re-injected at intervals when the patient could not resist doing things, which affected the facets.

Those who have described the hereditary spastic paraplegia, almost 130 years ago, have mentioned cases where retina, ophthalmic and auditory nerves were affected. These cases could well be facet syndromes. Eyes and auditory nerve are potential targets for any facet joint to attack since they belong to systems, which collaborate with the balance center. Their vasomotor centers are vulnerable to suffering facets.

In the presented case the vasomotor center, which responded to the facet triggering belongs to the locomotor system and the vessels affected were nutrient arteries of the corticospinal tract. On a relapse, it might be the vasomotor center of either the ophthalmic or the auditory system the one that might be triggered. Then, the facet's problem would be projected as an eye or ear problem. According to this concept the coincidence of paraplegia with blindness or deafness, reported in the original papers, could be irrelevant to hereditary factors. They could well be manifestations in sequence of the same facet syndrome.

The reason this spastic paraparesis case was recognized as a facet syndrome was its positive response to a facet treatment. The concept adopted for this case study is that suffering proprioceptors of lumbar facet joints were the triggering factor and the damage inflicted concerned the vascular supply of the corticospinal tract. This is the explanation the author could give in order to understand how he helped this patient. What he had to accept was that the triggering factor, which ever it is, was acting through lumbar facet joints.

This patient reminded him a few similar cases from the past. One of them concerns a patient visited at home five years earlier than the one described above for a low back pain which was going on and off parallel with a spastic paraparesis along a period of ten years. The patient could move around with the help of a wheelchair. He was seen again twice at the author's surgery for a relapse of the low back pain not on a wheelchair but walking with the aid of a stick. The patient's belief was that the paravertebral injections were those, which apart from the low back pain had helped spasticity to subside.

This was something, which at that time the author could not understand and let it pass. Evidently he had failed to correlate this patient's low back pain with his neurological problem until he came across the case described above. In this particular case the relapse of the orthopaedic problem was appearing parallel with a deterioration of spasticity and weakness of the legs. It was like two facet syndromes were running parallel, one displaying the skeletal problem through pain sensors as a low back pain and the other the neurologic one through proprioceptors, increasing spasticity and muscular weakness. In retrospect, the two different clinical conditions on this patient were accepted as different manifestations of the same facet syndrome.

Abdomen (General Surgery, Gastroenterology, Urology, Gynecology)

Abdomen is an area where proprioceptors of the lower thoracic and lumbar facets can also play around. General surgeons, gastroenterologists, urologists and gynecologists suspect that some of their problems start from the spine. Doctors seldom palpate their patient's spine unless they know what to look for. They are not few the cases where the thoracolumbar facets of a scoliotic curve have led to unnecessary cholecystectomies.

Meteorism

A thoracolumbar scoliotic curve was finally found to be the reason of the persisting meteorism of a general surgeon's secretary. Ogilvie's syndrome was among the possibilities. The paravertebral injections were those, which finally helped. A decent office chair was the remedy, which helped the patient.

Irritable Bowel

It was observed while treating facet syndromes on patients whose chronic problem was the irritable bowel that the symptoms, which characterize this entity, were occasionally retreating. These patients usually knew that psychological stress could affect their gastroenterological problem but they had never correlated it with the spine problem they had.

This subject is obviously out of an orthopaedic surgeon's scope but the temptation of mentioning it could not be avoided.

Testicle Pain

A young man, almost 40, appeared one day escorted by his physiotherapist for a persisting low back pain, which was radiating down the anterolateral side of his thigh. They were both motocross bike fans. It was the physiotherapist's suggestion to visit the orthopaedic surgeon after his efforts to help his friend came to a halt. He was wondering if an injection could finally help him.

The palpation revealed a muscular spasm and tenderness at the left of the spine, at the L2 to L4 level where the X-Ray films showed a very slight thoracolumbar curve. The patient was questioned if this pain had any radiation to the genitalia. His instant reaction was to turn towards the physiotherapist who promptly defended himself by saying: "I didn't mention anything". As they explained, he had been admitted urgently two weeks earlier in a private nursing home with an acute pain to his left testicle. All tests done proved nothing. Pain subsided gradually with sedatives. On the fifth day he was discharged with no diagnosis and having to pay a heavy bill for the thorough investigation he was submitted to. Injecting the tender lumbar facets his problem was solved.

Surgeons in general are aware that lumbar spine is often the origin of a testicle pain but they seldom ask the patient to turn over to examine his back. They most probably are not quite sure what to look for and not certain of how to proceed afterwards.

The After Intubation Syndromes

The hyperextension of the cervical spine, while the anesthetist tries to intubate a patient with stiff neck, might be followed by unexpected postoperative problems. Brachialgia is one of them. The surgeon is the one who is puzzled when he comes to face it. Most anesthetists are aware that this happens. Questioning the patients for any cervical problems they have, before putting them to sleep, and respecting the spine while intubating the patient, helps them avoid creating postoperative problems of this kind.

Rheumatoid Arthritis

Rheumatoid arthritis is a collagen disease and as such the rheumatologist is the right one to treat. The orthopaedic surgeon may be involved when there is need for surgical intervention to help with deformities. Quite often, he is approached by rheumatoid patients, to provide help for some kind of pain. He can do it as long as he does not interfere with the treatment regime the patient is already on.

Injecting a painful joint and the spine when facet involvement was suspected, although this was done to provide temporary relief, it was observed that quite often the response was not temporary at all. It probably concerned cases for which the term "pseudo rheumatism" was a convenient one to clinicians who were unaware of the existence of facet syndromes.

In cases of ankylosing spondylitis, a relapse of spinal pain does not always mean an exacerbation of the disease itself. A single injection has provided in many occasions relief for long periods. A rheumatoid patient can present, parallel to his disease, a facet problem too. Such cases are not a rarity and can be wrongly conceived as a relapse of the disease.

The author's impression is that he has helped rheumatoid patients to escape the joint deformities by injecting the suffering joints locally on each recurrence. This was done parallel to the regimen the patient was already on and apart of saving the joints helped the rheumatologist to keep the maintenance dose to the lowest possible level.

Radiculitis

Radiculitis is a term, which the author never understood. All cases he came across been previously diagnosed as such, responded when treated as facet syndromes. Radiculitis due to viruses, as in the case of Herpes, make their entrance in a more rowdy way. There has been an abuse, incriminating viruses for a lot of neuropathies. The facet joints could rightly claim to have a share on their etiology.

TREATMENT

The paravertebral injection was the method, which the author used to treat the facet syndromes. The usual number of weekly sessions was up to three. The second and third were following when the improvement after the first one was partial only.

These injections have nothing in common with the epidural or the transforaminal ones. One is not entering the spine canal, neither is approaching nerve roots. He has only to reach the posterolateral aspect of the facet joints. A disposable syringe of 5ml with a needle 21g and 1.5" long was the size, which proved safer in the author's hands while treating the cervical spine. Longer needles are occasionally needed when treating the lumbar facets of an obese patient.

Mixing a low absorption cortisone preparation with a local anesthetic in the same syringe was not found harmful for any of the thousands of patients treated this way. Doing it separately, one would never be certain if cortisone had reached the target. It is the local anesthetic the one, which provides this information when mixed with cortisone. Diabetic patients should get advice first by their own physician before starting this treatment.

Treating a facet syndrome, one accepts that he is handling a mechanically induced disorder. Apart of trauma, mechanical strain on facet joints is usually a factor. Questioning the patient, one tries to find out what is the real cause. Once he has done it, it is crucial to make it clear to his patient that he should not expect any improvement from any kind of treatment unless is ready to help by reducing strain and avoiding actions which have led to that. The patient should also understand that the improvement of the first days is only the announcement that healing has started. A few weeks of further care by the patient himself is imperative.

At the early stage of the disease, when symptoms start as mere smoke signals, which is a local or radiating pain, the infiltration of the facet joints alone is enough. When these signals have been ignored repeatedly, for weeks or even months then the vasomotor centers proceed with sacrifices. This is the time when peripheral vessels, nerves and organs or structures of the deep fascia start being affected. At this stage a peripheral problem is added. Although it is the facets that have started it, injecting them only, is not enough. The peripheral problem should be treated too with local injections or otherwise. This treatment cannot be much of help when irreversible tissue changes have affected these organs. Soft tissue therapists can prove much more effective with their clients if some kind of facet treatment has timely been provided to these patients before they have reached them.

The injection treatment is an aggressive process and certainly not free of risks. It suits more to surgically trained doctors who are familiar with handling emergencies. Injecting the cervical spine, a fainting episode is a condition, which one must be ready to face. One injects nothing to nobody without having available soluble cortisone for IV administration if needed.

71

Questioning for allergies and fainting episodes is imperative. Allergy to a local anesthetic, although rare, was the real nightmare through all these years of practice. With time, this incidence becomes a rarity since experience helps one to suspect these cases and handle carefully a patient who is prone to react badly. Anxiety is an alarm sign. It is increasing the patient's reactions. Flushing of face is occasionally met especially on women. This appears one or two days after and lasts another couple of days. A usual sedative is helpful for this to subside soon. A temporary rise of the white cell count might rarely appear. Suction before injecting is imperative.

Surgical imaging devices are terrifying the patient. Although useful at the beginning to help the injector find his target, they are time consuming and gradually prove to be less necessary. They may be helpful if the injector is certain which are the facets that need infiltration. The author never was. They are usually more than one.

An old standing stenosis of a disk space does not always mean that this is the suffering level. The stiffness of that space is often compensated by extra work at the above or lower level. It may be the suffering facets are hiding there. X-Rays and MRI are not of much help. It is the pain reaction to the injected fluid the one which can pinpoint them. They cannot be missed. Facets from upper or lower levels were often found to react this way. This means that the needle had to move up and down searching for them. When one has reached the point not to depend on localizing devices then the injecting process is much simplified and more easily accepted by the patient.

With the patient sitting on a couch, it takes no more than half a minute for each side of the cervical spine to be injected. This is actually the maximum time the patient can easily endure. The patient will state to his doctor, straight after being injected, that something has changed. This is a partial or full relief of pain. The insertion of the needle is not painful; it is the pressure of the injected fluid that hurts when the needle has reached the suffering joint. If the patient will thank on his leave the doctor for not having hurt him, this means that he has probably missed the target. With time and improvement of the target tracing ability, one finds out that smaller doses of the medicament can bring equally good results.

Treating the facet syndromes one hardly feels that he masters the game. Some facet joints might keep escaping. The second appointment is the one, which helps him find out. Not infrequently one comes to realize that the result is better when he has a reason to inject also facets from the opposite side. Although this may not be understandable, it happens.

Temporary loss of stability is common when injecting the cervical spine. This is more intense when one has to inject both sides at a time. It is the local anesthetic the one that puts out of action the balance proprioceptors. It takes ten to fifteen minutes for this function to be regained. The patient is not allowed to leave the surgery till he feels confident he can walk steadily.

What should be stressed is that one never injects cortisone if he suspects infection. This will fulminate it. The surgical field of an arthroplasty is a forbidden place too. Injecting there could prove disastrous if any non-detectable low-grade infection exists. The routine lab and X-R tests provide some protection from mistakes. One should also be on alert for a possible metastatic disease.

Patients with focusing problems are prone to develop a facet syndrome. An intermediate pair of eyeglasses is most important for computer users. Multifocal glasses are usually aggravating the problem instead of helping it. They achieve focusing by extending the neck.

The question which will not stop demanding an answer is: "who is to treat these syndromes: a naive artist or the specialists to whom these cases belong?" For the time being it is the one who knows how to do it properly.

RESISTANCE TO CHANGE

G etting familiar with the spine approach is essential in order to diagnose and treat a facet syndrome. Most doctors are not; neither encouraged to learn how to do it properly. Apart of spine surgeons, hardly any of the specialists involved are familiar with this process. The Anesthetists are an exception but are completely irrelevant to any of these clinical entities. This lack of familiarity with the spine approach is one of the reasons why medical practitioners are hesitant to get acquainted with these syndromes. Specialists with surgical training could easily get familiar but the rest will need help, on the start at least, by a spine surgeon. The advanced specialization has increased the difficulty in recognizing the cross medical field relationships. Medical practitioners feel more secure confining themselves in narrow parts of their own specialty trying to be good in that. Their ability to understand medicine as a whole, is steadily decreasing.

On the other hand the legal framework is not encouraging increased associated risks. As a result, although research is driving strong, the academic people have not encouraged the clinical venture in fields where they never felt safe enough. The approach of spine, especially in the cervical area is certainly an aggressive process in the same sense any surgical intervention is. Medicine was never halted by difficulties of this kind. The progress in understanding the facet syndromes, apart of providing relief to a huge number of patients, will have an analogous impact on bringing down the cost of health services. This counts to billions $ or Euros yearly for some of them.

THE OVERALL COST OF FACET SYNDROMES

S uch a research on facet syndromes has not yet been carried out for the whole of them. What is available is scattered information on the financial cost of hip and knee OA together. What is known is that 2.5 million people are living to day in USA with total hip replacements. 1.4 million of them are women and 1.1 million are men. The estimation is that the number of operations is gradually increasing. Only 5% of the sufferers are undergoing surgery and the cost on health services counts to some billions. The cost of conservative treatment on the hole of sufferers, the loss of income and the burden on production is bringing the overall cost three times up.

Diseases have a diagnostic cost also. The loss of time is increasing it. Injecting the spine straight away after suspecting a facet syndrome is practically the first diagnostic step on this purely clinical entity and at the same time the start of treatment. This was the routine process each time the author was called to the outpatients or casualty department to examine patients of this kind. This tactic, solving in most cases the diagnostic problem from the start, was saving money too. Lab tests were ordered, when the improvement of the first few days did not last.

This tactic proved helpful with the private patients too. Proceeding straight away with injections it helped in handling them. They were cooperative from the start, since finding improvement early, they felt that what was left to them was to follow instructions only. Looking backwards to the number of cases, which have past by, the amount of money saved for both health system and patients should be a considerable one. Treating these cases effectively is the biggest money saver. A dozen at least of medical specialties have facet problems. Not knowing how to treat them properly, a huge social and financial cost is accumulated.

The overall cost of syndromes which concern orthopaedics, amounts to billions yearly. The social and financial cost of Sudeck's syndrome is also considerable. Spinal pain related to facet joints is what one comes across in everyday practice. It is the acquaintance of doctors with these syndromes what will finally help.

EPILOGUE

M edicine can only be learned in practice. This is true with other sciences too. No matter what one has been taught or studied, what remains is only what the author had the chance to come across, to diagnose and then treat. The information is transformed to knowledge only if it is applied and proved working.

What one has read in these pages is just information. It is the author's kind of information gained out of practice and shaped to a concept when he came to realize that effective alternative treatment exists for many obscure clinical conditions if one could look at them from a different angle. What will certainly be questioned are the explanations he provides. They could not be avoided. If they are sound theories or questionable interpretations is the least that meant for him. They were just created to help him understand the facts. The facts are the realization that treatment is available for more than thirty clinical entities, which cover more than twelve medical specialties. If this was a reality for him, why it should not be also reality for the rest. The right interpretations on subtle mechanisms involved will be found and given by researchers whom any practitioner respects. The practitioner's motivation hardly exceeds his need to be effective with his patients. The available time is hardly enough for them.

Nikolaos Giantsios

Diagnostic and therapeutic methods, simpler than those the author has applied, would certainly be great help to those who would try to verify and treat their own cases. Depending on naive artists to help them with the spine approach is hardly the solution. Changes take time on their way to realization. Facet syndromes cannot be the exception. They have to be understood first.

ABOUT THE AUTHOR

N ikolaos (Nikos) Giantsios was born in Thessaloniki in 1932 and was brought up in Kozani, the hometown of his parents.

He received his degree from the Medical School of the Aristoteleion University of Thessaloniki. His postgraduate training as an Orthopaedic surgeon lasted a total of six and a half years; eighteen months in Athens (Children Orthopaedic Hospital at Penteli) and five years through six hospitals in the United Kingdom from Feb 1962 to Feb 1967 (The Royal National Orthopedic Hospital London, The Royal Hospital Chesterfield, War Memorial Hospital Rhyl North Wales, The Agnes Hunt and Robert Jones Orthopaedic Hospital at Oswestry, South Mead & Cossham Memorial Hospitals in Bristol, and Barnsley Hospital for general and vascular surgery).

He has been practicing Orthopaedics in Thessaloniki since 1967. During the early period, parallel to private practice he held appointments as Consulting Orthopaedic Surgeon by the 1st Surgical University Clinic at the AHEPA hospital from 1967 to 1976 at a time when trauma in northern Greece was still in hands of general surgeons and from 1979 to 1986 as a consulting orthopaedic surgeon to the Theagenion Cancer Hospital of Thessaloniki involved in the diagnosis and treatment of bone tumors. From that time and on, when the newly applied in his country NHS demanded full time involvement, he decided to confine himself in private practice. This proved to be a decisive moment after which, self-determination and survival kept evolving in balance all the way after.

He has two grown up children, Konstantinos and Fotini, for which he is very proud. He stopped skiing at the age of 78 when his younger wife Olga wisely refused to follow him any longer down the red slopes. Now he enjoys hiking and gardening with her. Carpentry has always been a hobby. He still believes that a few glasses of wine can go a long way towards enriching and livening up a productive conversation.

INDEX

cortisone · 10, 24, 25, 28, 39, 41, 47, 59, 67, 68, 70

A

Abdomen · 62
acute deafness · 24, 25
adhesions · 6, 27, 28, 29, 46, 50, 52
ankylosing spondylitis · 65
ANS · 3, 5, 42, 43
arteritis · 25
auditory · 23, 25, 26, 61

B

blindness · 26, 61
blurred vision · 22
brachial neuralgia · 12, 16, 17, 18, 19, 20
brachial plexus · 16
brachialgia · 13

C

Cardiac arrhythmia · 20
catarrh · 13
causalgia · 13, 17, 19
chiropractor · 27
chiropractors · 27

D

Deep fascia · 6, 32, 68
demineralization · 45
dentists · 2
dizziness · 13, 21, 22, 24, 26
dysphagia · 18, 19

E

ear noises · 24
Ear pain · 13
ENT · 2, 5, 13, 14, 15, 24, 25, 26

F

facial palsy · 19
fainting episodes · 23, 69
fasciitis · 37
frozen shoulder · 46

R

retina detachment · 23
rhinorrhoea · 20
Rt. acetabular fossa · 50

S

sinusitis · 14
Sleep apnea · 21
SLR · 56
Sneezing attacks · 20
spondylolisthesis · 36, 55
stomatologist · 13
Sudeck · 11, 44, 45, 46, 75

T

temporal arteritis · 26

tender heel · 32, 37
tennis elbow · 5, 31
transient diplopia · 22
trigeminal neuralgia · 12, 14, 15,
17, 19
trochanter · 33, 49

V

vasa nervorum · 16, 56, 57
virus · 17, 24
vision · 3, 4, 5, 22, 23

W

Whiplash injuries · 26
whiplash injury · 27

Nikolaos Giantsios

Nikolaos Giantsios